GASTROPARESIS COOKBOOK FOR BEGINNERS

Easy-to-Prepare Meals, Delicious and Digestive-Friendly Cooking for Starters

Smart Desty

Table of Contents

INTRODUCTION

Despite being a widespread ailment, gastroparesis is frequently misdiagnosed and poorly understood. Gastroparesis, which is characterized by delayed stomach emptying, can make eating and digesting difficult on a regular basis. Experiencing symptoms like nausea, vomiting, bloating, and abdominal pain can have a substantial negative effect on one's quality of life and make it difficult to choose healthy foods. If you or a loved one is dealing with gastroparesis, this cookbook is meant to provide practical solutions and assistance to help control symptoms via nutrition.

When the vagus nerve, which regulates the muscles of the stomach, is damaged, the stomach's capacity to evacuate its contents is compromised, leading to gastroparesis. Many conditions, such as diabetes, surgery, or sometimes no apparent cause at all, can lead to this illness. From person to person, the severity of gastroparesis might differ significantly. For some, it may entail occasional discomfort, while for others, it can result in regular hospital visits and severe limitations on everyday activities.

Finding foods that are both healthy and easily digested is the main issue while dealing with gastroparesis. Foods that are hard to digest, heavy in fat, or both can make symptoms worse. A gastroparesis diet therefore focuses on choosing meals that are easy on the stomach, aid with digestion, and reduce discomfort.

Dietary Guidelines for Gastroparesis

Knowing which items to eat to improve digestion and reduce symptoms is essential while navigating a gastroparesis diet. Here are some essential guidelines to help you along:

1. Select Low-Fiber Foods: Fiber can be uncomfortable and difficult to digest, which can lead to bloating. To reduce your intake of fiber, go for well-cooked veggies and refined grains.

2. Emphasize Smooth and Soft Foods: It is simpler to digest soft foods. Include foods like smoothies, soups, and mashed potatoes in your meals.

3. Consume Light Meals Frequently: Big meals can cause the stomach to feel overfull and hinder digestion. Meals that are smaller and more frequent may be gentler on your system.

4. Select Lean Proteins: Choose lean proteins like tofu, fish, and chicken. Steer clear of fried and fatty meats as they can delay the emptying of the stomach.

5. Maintain Hydration: It's important to stay hydrated, but watch what kinds of drinks you drink. Steer clear of high-sugar and fizzy beverages as these can induce bloating.

6. Apply Mild Cooking Techniques: It is better to steam, bake, or boil rather than fry or grill. These techniques can aid in preserving the food's suppleness and digestion.

Guides for Cooking and Eating Well

A careful approach is needed while cooking for gastroparesis in order to make meals both enjoyable and manageable. The following advice can help you enjoy cooking and eating more comfortably:

1. Make a meal plan: Making a meal plan may keep you organized and guarantee that the right meals are always available. Make sure your snacks and meals follow the nutritional recommendations for gastroparesis.

2. Prepare in Advance: Take into account batch cooking or meal prep in advance. This might relieve you of the burden

of preparing meals every day and guarantee that you always have healthy options on hand.

3. Keep an eye on portion sizes: By preparing smaller servings, you may control how much you eat and avoid uncomfortable or full feelings.

4. Try Different Textures: Some gastroparesis sufferers discover that their symptoms might change depending on the texture of their meal. Try different combinations of finely chopped, blended, and pureed foods to find what suits you the best.

5. Listen to Your Body: Observe how various meals and foods make you feel. Adapt your diet to your own comfort levels and tolerance.

The Cookbook's Goal

This cookbook aims to present you with a range of flavorful and varied recipes that follow the recommendations for people with gastroparesis. Having gastroparesis in mind when cooking doesn't have to mean sacrificing flavor or appeal. Actually, the goal of this cookbook is to demonstrate that you can make tasty, filling meals that meet your unique dietary requirements.

Every meal has been meticulously crafted to fulfill the nutritional guidelines for gastroparesis while maintaining ease of preparation. You have a wide variety of meal ideas to pick from because we've included alternatives for breakfast, lunch, dinner, snacks, and desserts. Beginners will find it easier to handle the complexity of cooking for gastroparesis thanks to the dishes' straightforward and approachable style.

Although having gastroparesis can be difficult, you can control your symptoms and enhance your quality of life by following a healthy diet and cooking routine. This cookbook offers helpful, simple-to-follow recipes and advice to help make meal preparation a little less intimidating so that you can feel less alone on your journey. We hope that these dishes will not only satisfy your dietary requirements but also make mealtimes more enjoyable and fulfilling.

Thank you for selecting this cookbook as a source. I know you can handle gastroparesis confidently and find comfort in your meals if you have the necessary tools, patience, and inventiveness.

CHAPTER ONE: BREAKFAST RECIPES

Let's explore 15 breakfast recipes tailored for gastroparesis, with each recipe designed to be gentle on the stomach while providing essential nutrients.

1. Banana Oat Smoothie

Ingredients:

- 1 ripe banana

- 1/2 cup rolled oats

- 1/2 cup low-fat yogurt

- 1/2 cup almond milk (or any preferred low-fat milk)

- 1 tablespoon honey (optional)

Instructions:

1. Peel and slice the banana.

2. Combine all ingredients in a blender.

3. Blend until smooth and creamy.

4. Pour into a glass and serve immediately.

Prep Time: 5 minutes Cook Time: 0 minutes

Nutritional Composition (per serving):

Calories: 250| Protein: 8g | Carbohydrates: 45g

Fat: 4g | Fiber: 3g

2. Creamy Rice Porridge

Ingredients:

- 1/2 cup white rice

- 1 1/2 cups water

- 1 cup low-fat milk

- 1 tablespoon honey

- 1/4 teaspoon ground cinnamon

Instructions:

1. Rinse the rice under cold water.
2. In a saucepan, combine rice and water. Bring to a boil.
3. Reduce heat, cover, and simmer for 15 minutes.
4. Stir in milk, honey, and cinnamon. Cook for another 5 minutes, stirring occasionally.
5. Serve warm.

Prep Time: 5 minutes | Cook Time: 20 minutes

Nutritional Composition (per serving):

Calories: 220 | Protein: 7g | Carbohydrates: 40g

Fat: 3g | Fiber: 1g

3. Scrambled Eggs with Spinach

Ingredients:

- 2 large eggs

- 1/4 cup fresh spinach, finely chopped

- 1 tablespoon olive oil

- Salt to taste

Instructions:

1. Heat olive oil in a non-stick skillet over medium heat.

2. Whisk the eggs and add to the skillet.

3. Cook, stirring occasionally, until eggs start to set.

4. Add spinach and cook until eggs are fully set.

5. Season with salt to taste and serve.

Prep Time: 5 minutes | Cook Time: 5 minutes

Nutritional Composition (per serving):

Calories: 180 | Protein: 12g | Carbohydrates: 2g

Fat: 14g | Fiber: 1g

4. Apple Cinnamon Oatmeal

Ingredients:

- 1/2 cup rolled oats

- 1/2 cup diced apples (peeled)

- 1 cup water

- 1/2 cup low-fat milk

- 1/2 teaspoon ground cinnamon

Instructions:

1. In a saucepan, bring water to a boil.
2. Add oats and apples. Reduce heat and simmer for 5 minutes.
3. Stir in milk and cinnamon. Cook for another 5 minutes.
4. Serve warm.

Prep Time: 5 minutes | Cook Time: 10 minutes

Nutritional Composition (per serving):

Calories: 220 | Protein: 6g |Carbohydrates: 38g

Fat: 4g | Fiber: 3g

5. Yogurt with Honey and Berries

Ingredients:

- 1 cup low-fat yogurt

- 1 tablespoon honey

- 1/4 cup fresh berries (blueberries or raspberries)

Instructions:

1. Spoon yogurt into a bowl.

2. Drizzle honey on top.

3. Scatter berries over the yogurt.

4. Serve immediately.

Prep Time: 5 minutes   Cook Time: 0 minutes

Nutritional Composition (per serving):

Calories: 180 | Protein: 8g | Carbohydrates: 28g

Fat: 2g | Fiber: 2g

6. Creamy Pumpkin Soup

Ingredients:

- 1 cup canned pumpkin puree

- 1 cup low-sodium vegetable broth

- 1/2 cup low-fat milk

- 1/4 teaspoon ground ginger

- Salt to taste

Instructions:

1. In a saucepan, combine pumpkin puree and vegetable broth. Heat over medium heat.
2. Stir in milk and ginger. Cook until heated through.
3. Season with salt to taste and serve.

Prep Time: 5 minutes | Cook Time: 10 minutes

Nutritional Composition (per serving):

Calories: 120 | Protein: 4g

Carbohydrates: 20g | Fat: 2g | Fiber: 2g

7. Poached Eggs with Avocado

Ingredients:

- 2 large eggs

- 1/2 ripe avocado

- Salt and pepper to taste

Instructions:

1. Fill a saucepan with water and bring to a simmer.
2. Crack eggs into a small bowl, then gently slide them into the simmering water.
3. Cook for 3-4 minutes until whites are set but yolks are runny.
4. Remove eggs with a slotted spoon.
5. Slice avocado and serve with eggs.
6. Season with salt and pepper.

Prep Time: 5 minutes | Cook Time: 5 minutes

Nutritional Composition (per serving):

Calories: 230 | Protein: 12g |Carbohydrates: 12g

Fat: 18g | Fiber: 4g

8. Mashed Sweet Potatoes

Ingredients:

- 1 large sweet potato

- 1/4 cup low-fat milk

- 1 tablespoon butter

- Salt to taste

Instructions:

1. Peel and dice sweet potato. Boil in water until tender, about 15 minutes.
2. Drain and mash with a fork.
3. Stir in milk and butter until smooth.
4. Season with salt to taste and serve.

Prep Time: 10 minutes | Cook Time: 15 minutes

Nutritional Composition (per serving):

Calories: 180 | Protein: 2g |Carbohydrates: 40g

Fat: 4g | Fiber: 5g

9. Cottage Cheese with Fruit

Ingredients:

- 1 cup low-fat cottage cheese

- 1/2 cup diced peaches or pears (canned in juice, drained)

Instructions:

1. Spoon cottage cheese into a bowl.

2. Top with diced fruit.

3. Serve immediately.

Prep Time: 5 minutes | Cook Time: 0 minutes

Nutritional Composition (per serving):

Calories: 200 | Protein: 14g |Carbohydrates: 20g

Fat: 4g |Fiber: 2g

10. Baked Apples with Cinnamon

Ingredients:

- 2 medium apples, cored

- 2 tablespoons honey

- 1/2 teaspoon ground cinnamon

Instructions:

1. Preheat oven to 350°F (175°C).

2. Place apples in a baking dish.

3. Drizzle with honey and sprinkle with cinnamon.

4. Bake for 20 minutes until tender.

5. Serve warm.

Prep Time: 10 minutes | Cook Time: 20 minutes

Nutritional Composition (per serving):

Calories: 150 | Protein: 1g |Carbohydrates: 40g

Fat: 0g |Fiber: 5g

11. Quinoa Breakfast Bowl

Ingredients:

- 1/2 cup cooked quinoa

- 1/2 cup low-fat milk

- 1 tablespoon maple syrup

- 1/4 cup sliced bananas

Instructions:

1. Warm cooked quinoa in a bowl.

2. Stir in milk and maple syrup.

3. Top with sliced bananas.

4. Serve warm.

Prep Time: 5 minutes | Cook Time: 5 minutes

Nutritional Composition (per serving):

Calories: 220 |Protein: 7g |Carbohydrates: 38g

Fat: 4g |Fiber: 3g

12. Soft-Boiled Eggs with Toast

Ingredients:

- 2 large eggs

- 1 slice white bread

Instructions:

1. Boil water in a saucepan.

2. Gently add eggs and cook for 6-7 minutes for soft-boiled.

3. Remove eggs and place in cold water for a minute.

4. Toast the bread and cut into strips.

5. Peel and serve eggs with toast.

Prep Time: 5 minutes |Cook Time: 7 minutes

Nutritional Composition (per serving):

Calories: 250 |Protein: 13g |Carbohydrates: 20g

Fat: 14g |Fiber: 1g

13. Creamy Avocado Toast

Ingredients:

- 1 ripe avocado

- 1 slice white bread

- Salt and pepper to taste

Instructions:

1. Toast the bread.

2. Mash avocado in a bowl and season with salt and pepper.

3. Spread avocado mixture on the toasted bread.

4. Serve immediately.

Prep Time: 5 minutes | Cook Time: 5 minutes

Nutritional Composition (per serving):

Calories: 250 | Protein: 4g |Carbohydrates: 23g

Fat: 18g | Fiber: 5g

14. Smoothie with Spinach and Banana

Ingredients:

- 1 cup fresh spinach

- 1 banana

- 1/2 cup low-fat yogurt

- 1/2 cup apple juice

Instructions:

1. Place all ingredients in a blender.

2. Blend until smooth.

3. Pour into a glass and serve immediately.

Prep Time: 5 minutes

Cook Time: 0 minutes

Nutritional Composition (per serving):

Calories: 220

Protein: 8g

Carbohydrates: 40g

Fat: 2g

Fiber: 3g

15. Rice Pudding with Vanilla

Ingredients:

- 1/2 cup cooked white rice

- 1 cup low-fat milk

- 2 tablespoons sugar

- 1/2 teaspoon vanilla extract

Instructions:

1. In a saucepan, combine cooked rice and milk. Heat over medium heat.
2. Stir in sugar and vanilla extract.
3. Cook, stirring occasionally, until the mixture thickens.
4. Serve warm or chilled.

Prep Time: 5 minutes | Cook Time: 15 minutes

Nutritional Composition (per serving):

Calories: 200 | Protein: 6g |Carbohydrates: 35g

Fat: 4g |Fiber: 1g

These recipes are crafted to be gentle on the stomach while providing balanced nutrition. Feel free to adjust ingredients and seasonings based on personal tolerance and preferences.

CHAPTER TWO:

LUNCH RECIPES

Enjoy fifteen 15 lunch recipes designed for those with gastroparesis. Each recipe is crafted to be gentle on the stomach while providing balanced and nutritious options.

1. Creamy Chicken and Rice Soup

Ingredients:

- 1 cup cooked chicken breast, shredded
- 1/2 cup cooked white rice
- 2 cups low-sodium chicken broth
- 1/2 cup low-fat milk
- 1/4 cup finely chopped carrots
- 1 tablespoon olive oil

Instructions:

1. Heat olive oil in a pot over medium heat.
2. Add carrots and cook until soft, about 5 minutes.
3. Add chicken broth and bring to a boil.
4. Stir in shredded chicken and cooked rice. Simmer for 5 minutes.
5. Stir in milk and cook until heated through.
6. Serve warm.

Prep Time: 10 minutes | Cook Time: 15 minutes

Nutritional Composition (per serving):

Calories: 220 | Protein: 15g |Carbohydrates: 25g

Fat: 7g | Fiber: 1g

2. Mashed Sweet Potato and Chicken

Ingredients:

- 1 cup cooked, mashed sweet potatoes

- 1/2 cup cooked, shredded chicken breast

- 1/4 cup low-fat chicken broth

- 1 tablespoon olive oil

- Salt to taste

Instructions:

1. Heat olive oil in a skillet over medium heat.
2. Add shredded chicken and chicken broth. Cook until heated through.
3. Stir in mashed sweet potatoes until well combined.
4. Season with salt to taste and serve.

Prep Time: 5 minutes | Cook Time: 10 minutes

Nutritional Composition (per serving):

Calories: 270 | Protein: 20g | Carbohydrates: 30g

Fat: 10g | Fiber: 4g

3. Soft-Cooked Vegetable Soup

Ingredients:

- 1 cup diced potatoes

- 1/2 cup finely chopped carrots

- 1/2 cup finely chopped zucchini

- 2 cups low-sodium vegetable broth

- 1/4 cup low-fat milk

Instructions:

1. In a pot, combine potatoes, carrots, and vegetable broth.
2. Bring to a boil, then reduce heat and simmer until vegetables are tender, about 15 minutes.
3. Add zucchini and cook for another 5 minutes.
4. Stir in milk and serve warm.

Prep Time: 10 minutes | Cook Time: 20 minutes

Nutritional Composition (per serving):

Calories: 150 | Protein: 4g | Carbohydrates: 30g

Fat: 2g | Fiber: 4g

4. Baked Fish Fillet with Rice

Ingredients:

- 1 fish fillet (such as cod or tilapia)

- 1/2 cup cooked white rice

- 1 tablespoon olive oil

- 1/2 teaspoon dried herbs (such as dill or thyme)

- Salt to taste

Instructions:

1. Preheat oven to 375°F (190°C).
2. Place fish fillet on a baking sheet, drizzle with olive oil, and sprinkle with dried herbs and salt.
3. Bake for 15-20 minutes, until the fish is cooked through and flakes easily.
4. Serve with cooked rice.

Prep Time: 10 minutes | Cook Time: 20 minutes

Nutritional Composition (per serving):

Calories: 220 | Protein: 20g |Carbohydrates: 22g

Fat: 7g | Fiber: 1g

5. Creamy Spinach and Egg Salad

Ingredients:

- 2 hard-boiled eggs, chopped

- 1/2 cup fresh spinach, finely chopped

- 2 tablespoons low-fat Greek yogurt

- 1 teaspoon lemon juice

- Salt to taste

Instructions:

1. In a bowl, combine chopped eggs and spinach.

2. Stir in Greek yogurt and lemon juice.

3. Season with salt to taste and serve.

Prep Time: 10 minutes

Cook Time: 0 minutes

Nutritional Composition (per serving):

Calories: 150 | Protein: 12g | Carbohydrates: 4g

Fat: 10g | Fiber: 1g

6. Quinoa and Soft Veggie Salad

Ingredients:

- 1 cup cooked quinoa

- 1/2 cup cooked, diced carrots

- 1/2 cup cooked, diced zucchini

- 1 tablespoon olive oil

- Salt to taste

Instructions:

1. In a bowl, combine cooked quinoa, carrots, and zucchini.

2. Drizzle with olive oil and season with salt.

3. Toss gently and serve.

Prep Time: 10 minutes

Cook Time: 0 minutes

Nutritional Composition (per serving):

Calories: 220 | Protein: 6g | Carbohydrates: 32g

Fat: 8g | Fiber: 4g

7. Soft-Cooked Chicken and Carrot Stew

Ingredients:

- 1 cup cooked, shredded chicken breast

- 1/2 cup diced carrots

- 1 cup low-sodium chicken broth

- 1/4 cup low-fat milk

- 1 tablespoon olive oil

Instructions:

1. Heat olive oil in a pot over medium heat.

2. Add carrots and cook until soft, about 5 minutes.

3. Add chicken broth and bring to a boil.

4. Stir in shredded chicken and simmer for 5 minutes.

5. Stir in milk and serve.

Prep Time: 10 minutes | Cook Time: 10 minutes

Nutritional Composition (per serving):

Calories: 250 | Protein: 20g | Carbohydrates: 20g

Fat: 10g | Fiber: 2g

8. Soft-Boiled Egg with Mashed Sweet Potatoes

Ingredients:

- 1 large egg

- 1/2 cup mashed sweet potatoes

- Salt to taste

Instructions:

1. Boil water in a saucepan.

2. Add egg and cook for 6-7 minutes for a soft-boiled egg.

3. Peel the egg and serve with mashed sweet potatoes.

4. Season with salt to taste.

Prep Time: 5 minutes | Cook Time: 7 minutes

Nutritional Composition (per serving):

Calories: 200 | Protein: 11g | Carbohydrates: 25g

Fat: 7g | Fiber: 3g

9. Creamy Cauliflower Soup

Ingredients:

- 1 cup cauliflower florets

- 1 cup low-sodium vegetable broth

- 1/2 cup low-fat milk

- 1 tablespoon olive oil

- Salt to taste

Instructions:

1. In a pot, combine cauliflower and vegetable broth. Bring to a boil.
2. Reduce heat and simmer until cauliflower is tender, about 15 minutes.
3. Blend until smooth using an immersion blender.
4. Stir in milk and olive oil. Season with salt and serve.

Prep Time: 10 minutes | Cook Time: 15 minutes

Nutritional Composition (per serving):

Calories: 140 | Protein: 4g | Carbohydrates: 20g

Fat: 6g | Fiber: 3g

10. Turkey and Avocado Wrap

Ingredients:

- 2 slices lean turkey breast

- 1/4 avocado, sliced

- 1 whole wheat wrap (or white wrap if preferred)

- 1 tablespoon low-fat Greek yogurt

Instructions:

1. Spread Greek yogurt on the wrap.

2. Layer turkey slices and avocado on the wrap.

3. Roll up and slice in half. Serve immediately.

Prep Time: 5 minutes

Cook Time: 0 minutes

Nutritional Composition (per serving):

Calories: 200 | Protein: 15g | Carbohydrates: 20g

Fat: 8g | Fiber: 4g

11. Baked Sweet Potato with Greek Yogurt

Ingredients:

- 1 medium sweet potato

- 1/4 cup low-fat Greek yogurt

- 1 tablespoon honey

- Cinnamon to taste

Instructions:

1. Preheat oven to 400°F (200°C).
2. Pierce sweet potato with a fork and bake for 45 minutes until tender.
3. Cut open and top with Greek yogurt, honey, and cinnamon.
4. Serve warm.

Prep Time: 5 minutes | Cook Time: 45 minutes

Nutritional Composition (per serving):

Calories: 230 | Protein: 8g | Carbohydrates: 45g

Fat: 2g | Fiber: 5g

12. Spinach and Cottage Cheese Stuffed Bell Peppers

Ingredients:

- 2 bell peppers, halved and seeded

- 1/2 cup low-fat cottage cheese

- 1/2 cup fresh spinach, chopped

- 1 tablespoon olive oil

Instructions:

1. Preheat oven to 375°F (190°C).

2. In a bowl, mix cottage cheese and spinach.

3. Stuff bell pepper halves with the mixture.

4. Place in a baking dish and drizzle with olive oil.

5. Bake for 20 minutes until peppers are tender.

Prep Time: 10 minutes | Cook Time: 20 minutes

Nutritional Composition (per serving):

Calories: 150 | Protein: 12g | Carbohydrates: 15g

Fat: 6g | Fiber: 3g

13. Soft-Cooked Pasta with Tomato Sauce

Ingredients:

- 1 cup cooked pasta (such as macaroni or small shells)

- 1/2 cup low-sodium tomato sauce

- 1 tablespoon olive oil

- 1/4 teaspoon dried basil

Instructions:

1. Heat tomato sauce and olive oil in a saucepan.

2. Stir in cooked pasta and cook until heated through.

3. Sprinkle with dried basil and serve.

Prep Time: 5 minutes | Cook Time: 5 minutes

Nutritional Composition (per serving):

Calories: 220 | Protcin: 6g | Carbohydrates: 35g

Fat: 7g | Fiber: 2g

14. Creamy Lentil Soup

Ingredients:

- 1 cup cooked lentils

- 1 cup low-sodium vegetable broth

- 1/2 cup low-fat milk

- 1/4 teaspoon ground cumin

- Salt to taste

Instructions:

1. In a pot, combine cooked lentils and vegetable broth. Heat until simmering.
2. Stir in milk and ground cumin.
3. Blend until smooth using an immersion blender.
4. Season with salt and serve.

Prep Time: 10 minutes | Cook Time: 15 minutes

Nutritional Composition (per serving):

Calories: 180 | Protein: 8g | Carbohydrates: 30g

Fat: 3g | Fiber: 7g

15. Soft-Cooked Chicken and Rice Casserole

Ingredients:

- 1 cup cooked, shredded chicken breast

- 1/2 cup cooked white rice

- 1/2 cup low-fat milk

- 1/4 cup low-sodium chicken broth

- 1/4 cup finely chopped peas

Instructions:

1. Preheat oven to 350°F (175°C).
2. In a baking dish, combine chicken, rice, milk, chicken broth, and peas.
3. Bake for 20 minutes, until heated through.
4. Serve warm.

Prep Time: 10 minutes | Cook Time: 20 minutes

Nutritional Composition (per serving):

Calories: 250 | Protein: 20g | Carbohydrates: 30g

Fat: 6g | Fiber: 3g

CHAPTER THREE:
DINNER RECIPES

Healthy dinner suitable for your stomach health; enjoy these fifteen recipes:

1. Baked Chicken Breast with Mashed Potatoes

Ingredients:

- 1 chicken breast

- 1 tablespoon olive oil

- 1/2 teaspoon dried thyme

- 1 cup mashed potatoes (made with low-fat milk and butter)

- Salt to taste

Instructions:

1. Preheat oven to 375°F (190°C).

2. Rub the chicken breast with olive oil, thyme, and salt.

3. Bake for 25-30 minutes, or until cooked through.

4. Serve with mashed potatoes.

Prep Time: 10 minutes | Cook Time: 30 minutes

Nutritional Composition (per serving):

Calories: 300 | Protein: 25g | Carbohydrates: 30g

Fat: 10g | Fiber: 3g

2. Soft-Cooked Carrot and Potato Stew

Ingredients:

- 1 cup diced potatoes

- 1 cup diced carrots

- 2 cups low-sodium vegetable broth

- 1/4 cup low-fat milk

- 1 tablespoon olive oil

Instructions:

1. Heat olive oil in a pot over medium heat.
2. Add potatoes and carrots. Cook for 5 minutes.
3. Add vegetable broth and bring to a boil.
4. Reduce heat and simmer until vegetables are tender, about 15 minutes.
5. Stir in milk and serve.

Prep Time: 10 minutes | Cook Time: 20 minutes

Nutritional Composition (per serving):

Calories: 180 |Protein: 4g | Carbohydrates: 35g

Fat: 5g | Fiber: 5g

3. Tender Turkey Meatballs with Rice

Ingredients:

- 1/2 pound ground turkey

- 1/4 cup cooked white rice

- 1 egg white

- 1/4 cup breadcrumbs

- 1/4 teaspoon dried oregano

- Salt to taste

Instructions:

1. Preheat oven to 375°F (190°C).
2. Mix ground turkey, rice, egg white, breadcrumbs, oregano, and salt.
3. Form into meatballs and place on a baking sheet.
4. Bake for 20 minutes or until cooked through.
5. Serve warm.

Prep Time: 10 minutes | Cook Time: 20 minutes

Nutritional Composition (per serving, 4 meatballs):

Calories: 250 | Protein: 22g | Carbohydrates: 20g

Fat: 10g | Fiber: 2g

4. Baked Cod with Steamed Green Beans

Ingredients:

- 1 cod fillet

- 1 tablespoon olive oil

- 1/2 teaspoon dried parsley

- 1 cup green beans, trimmed

- Salt to taste

Instructions:

1. Preheat oven to 375°F (190°C).

2. Rub cod fillet with olive oil, parsley, and salt.

3. Bake for 15-20 minutes until fish flakes easily.

4. Steam green beans for 5 minutes until tender.

5. Serve cod with green beans.

Prep Time: 10 minutes | Cook Time: 20 minutes

Nutritional Composition (per serving):

Calories: 200 | Protein: 22g | Carbohydrates: 15g

Fat: 8g | Fiber: 4g

5. Creamy Chicken and Mushroom Bake

Ingredients:

- 1 cup cooked chicken breast, diced

- 1/2 cup sliced mushrooms

- 1/2 cup low-fat cream of chicken soup

- 1/4 cup low-fat milk

- 1 tablespoon olive oil

Instructions:

1. Preheat oven to 350°F (175°C).
2. In a baking dish, combine chicken, mushrooms, cream of chicken soup, and milk.
3. Drizzle with olive oil and bake for 20 minutes.
4. Serve warm.

Prep Time: 10 minutes | Cook Time: 20 minutes

Nutritional Composition (per serving):

Calories: 250 | Protein: 20g | Carbohydrates: 15g

Fat: 12g | Fiber: 2g

6. Soft-Cooked Spinach and Ricotta Stuffed Shells

Ingredients:

- 6 large pasta shells

- 1/2 cup ricotta cheese

- 1/2 cup fresh spinach, finely chopped

- 1/2 cup low-fat tomato sauce

- 1/4 cup shredded mozzarella cheese

Instructions:

1. Preheat oven to 375°F (190°C).
2. Cook pasta shells according to package instructions.
3. Mix ricotta and spinach. Stuff mixture into pasta shells.
4. Place stuffed shells in a baking dish and cover with tomato sauce.
5. Sprinkle with mozzarella cheese and bake for 20 minutes.

Prep Time: 15 minutes | Cook Time: 20 minutes

Nutritional Composition (per serving, 3 shells):

Calories: 220 | Protein: 12g | Carbohydrates: 30g

Fat: 8g | Fiber: 2g

7. Baked Turkey and Veggie Patties

Ingredients:

- 1/2 pound ground turkey

- 1/2 cup finely grated carrots

- 1/4 cup finely chopped zucchini

- 1 egg white

- 1/4 cup breadcrumbs

- 1 tablespoon olive oil

Instructions:

1. Preheat oven to 375°F (190°C).
2. Mix ground turkey, carrots, zucchini, egg white, and breadcrumbs.
3. Form into patties and place on a baking sheet.
4. Bake for 20 minutes or until cooked through.

Prep Time: 10 minutes | Cook Time: 20 minutes

Nutritional Composition (per serving, 2 patties):

Calories: 230 | Protein: 20g | Carbohydrates: 15g

Fat: 12g | Fiber: 2g

8. Creamy Butternut Squash Soup

Ingredients:

- 2 cups peeled and cubed butternut squash

- 1 cup low-sodium vegetable broth

- 1/2 cup low-fat milk

- 1 tablespoon olive oil

- Salt and pepper to taste

Instructions:

1. Heat olive oil in a pot over medium heat.
2. Add butternut squash and vegetable broth. Bring to a boil.
3. Reduce heat and simmer until squash is tender, about 15 minutes.
4. Blend until smooth. Stir in milk and season with salt and pepper.

Prep Time: 10 minutes | Cook Time: 15 minutes

Nutritional Composition (per serving):

Calories: 160 | Protein: 4g | Carbohydrates: 30g

Fat: 6g | Fiber: 4g

9. Soft-Cooked Salmon with Steamed Asparagus

Ingredients:

- 1 salmon fillet

- 1 tablespoon olive oil

- 1/2 teaspoon dried dill

- 1 cup asparagus spears, trimmed

- Salt to taste

Instructions:

1. Preheat oven to 375°F (190°C).

2. Rub salmon fillet with olive oil, dill, and salt.

3. Bake for 15 minutes or until salmon flakes easily.

4. Steam asparagus for 5 minutes until tender.

5. Serve salmon with asparagus.

Prep Time: 10 minutes | Cook Time: 15 minutes

Nutritional Composition (per serving):

Calories: 220 | Protein: 22g | Carbohydrates: 10g

Fat: 12g | Fiber: 4g

10. Soft-Cooked Rice with Chicken and Peas

Ingredients:

- 1 cup cooked white rice

- 1/2 cup cooked, diced chicken breast

- 1/4 cup cooked peas

- 1/4 cup low-fat chicken broth

- 1 tablespoon olive oil

Instructions:

1. Heat olive oil in a pan over medium heat.

2. Add chicken and peas, then stir in chicken broth.

3. Cook until heated through, about 5 minutes.

4. Stir in cooked rice and serve.

Prep Time: 5 minutes | Cook Time: 5 minutes

Nutritional Composition (per serving):

Calories: 230 | Protein: 15g | Carbohydrates: 35g

Fat: 8g | Fiber: 2g

11. Soft-Cooked Vegetable and Quinoa Pilaf

Ingredients:

- 1/2 cup cooked quinoa

- 1/2 cup finely diced carrots

- 1/2 cup finely diced zucchini

- 1/2 cup low-sodium vegetable broth

- 1 tablespoon olive oil

Instructions:

1. Heat olive oil in a skillet over medium heat.
2. Add carrots and zucchini, cook until soft, about 5 minutes.
3. Stir in cooked quinoa and vegetable broth. Heat until warmed through.
4. Serve warm.

Prep Time: 10 minutes | Cook Time: 10 minutes

Nutritional Composition (per serving):

Calories: 210 | Protein: 6g | Carbohydrates: 35g

Fat: 8g | Fiber: 4g

12. Tender Beef Stroganoff with Noodles

Ingredients:

- 1/2 pound beef sirloin, thinly sliced

- 1/2 cup low-fat sour cream

- 1/2 cup low-sodium beef broth

- 1/4 cup finely chopped onions

- 1 cup cooked egg noodles

Instructions:

1. Heat a pan over medium heat and cook onions until translucent.
2. Add beef slices and cook until browned.
3. Stir in beef broth and simmer for 5 minutes.
4. Stir in sour cream and cook until heated through.
5. Serve over cooked egg noodles.

Prep Time: 10 minutes | Cook Time: 15 minutes

Nutritional Composition (per serving):

Calories: 290 | Protein: 22g | Carbohydrates: 30g

Fat: 10g | Fiber: 2g

13. Soft-Cooked Eggplant and Tomato Casserole

Ingredients:

- 1 cup diced eggplant

- 1 cup diced tomatoes

- 1/2 cup low-fat mozzarella cheese

- 1 tablespoon olive oil

- Salt and pepper to taste

Instructions:

1. Preheat oven to 375°F (190°C).

2. In a baking dish, layer eggplant and tomatoes.

3. Drizzle with olive oil and season with salt and pepper.

4. Sprinkle with mozzarella cheese and bake for 20 minutes.

Prep Time: 10 minutes | Cook Time: 20 minutes

Nutritional Composition (per serving):

Calories: 180 | Protein: 10g | Carbohydrates: 20g

Fat: 8g | Fiber: 4g

14. Creamy Chicken and Spinach Pasta

Ingredients:

- 1 cup cooked pasta (such as penne)

- 1/2 cup cooked, diced chicken breast

- 1/2 cup fresh spinach, chopped

- 1/2 cup low-fat cream sauce

- 1 tablespoon olive oil

Instructions:

1. Heat olive oil in a pan over medium heat.

2. Add chicken and spinach, cook until spinach is wilted.

3. Stir in cream sauce and heat until warmed through.

4. Toss with cooked pasta and serve.

Prep Time: 10 minutes | Cook Time: 10 minutes

Nutritional Composition (per serving):

Calories: 250 | Protein: 20g |Carbohydrates: 25g

Fat: 8g | Fiber: 3g

15. Soft-Cooked Chicken and Sweet Potato Curry

Ingredients:

- 1 cup cooked, diced chicken breast

- 1 cup diced sweet potatoes

- 1/2 cup low-fat coconut milk

- 1 tablespoon curry powder

- 1 tablespoon olive oil

Instructions:

1. Heat olive oil in a pan over medium heat.

2. Add sweet potatoes and cook until tender, about 10 minutes.

3. Stir in chicken, coconut milk, and curry powder. Cook until heated through.

4. Serve warm.

Prep Time: 10 minutes | Cook Time: 15 minutes

Nutritional Composition (per serving):

Calories: 290 | Protein: 20g | Carbohydrates: 35g

Fat: 10g | Fiber: 4g

CHAPTER FOUR:

SNACKS AND DESSERTS

These 15 dishes for snacks and desserts are geared at those who have gastroparesis. Every meal is designed to satisfy your appetites for both sweet and savory foods without putting too much strain on your stomach.

1. Berry and yogurt smoothie

Components:

- Half a cup of low-fat yogurt

- 1/2 cup of mixed berries, including raspberries, strawberries, and blueberries

- One half banana

- Half a cup of apple juice

Guidelines:

1. Fill a blender with all the ingredients.

2. Process until smooth.

3. Immediately serve after pouring into a glass.

Time to Prepare: 5 minutes; Time to Cook: 0 minutes

Nutritional Value (per portion):
220 calories | 8g of protein | 40g of carbohydrates
Fat (2 grams) | 4g of fiber

2. Cinnamon-infused Applesauce

Components:

- One cup of plain applesauce

- Half a teaspoon of ground cinnamon

Guidelines:

1. Stir cinnamon into applesauce.

2. You can serve it cold or room temperature.

Time to Prepare: 2 minutes; Time to Cook: 0 minutes

Nutritional Value (per portion):

100 calories | Protein: nil | 26g of carbohydrates

Fat: 0 grams | 2g of fiber

3. Pear Compote, Soft-Cooked

Components:

- 1 tablespoon honey

- 1/4 cup water

- 2 ripe pears, peeled and chopped

Guidelines:

1. In a saucepan, mix pears, water, and honey.

2. Simmer for about ten minutes on low heat, or until pears are tender.

3. You can serve it cold or heated.

Cooking Time: 10 minutes

Nutritional Composition (per serving): 150 calories | Protein: nil | 38g of carbohydrates | Fat: 0 grams | 4g of fiber

4. Smoothie with bananas and peanut butter

Components:

- One banana

- One spoonful of peanut butter, smooth

- Half a cup of skim milk

- Half a cup of ice cubes

Guidelines:

1. Fill a blender with all the ingredients.

2. Process until smooth.

3. Transfer into a glass for serving.

Time to Prepare: 5 minutes; Time to Cook: 0 minutes

Nutritional Value (per portion):

250 calories | 8g of protein | 35g of carbohydrates

10g of fat | 4g of fiber

5. Honey-yogurt Parfait

Components:

– 1/2 cup Greek yogurt with reduced fat

- 1/4 cup smashed graham crackers

- 1 tablespoon honey

Guidelines:

1. Arrange honey and yogurt in a bowl.

2. Add crushed graham crackers on top.

3. Present right away.

Time to Prepare: 5 minutes; Time to Cook: 0 minutes

Nutritional Value (per portion):

200 calories | 10g of protein | 30g of carbohydrates

6g of fat | 1g of fiber

6. Cinnamon-Scented Soft-Cooked Apple Slices

Components:

- One peeled and sliced apple

- One-half teaspoon of ground cinnamon

- One tablespoon of water

Guidelines:

1. Put apple slices in a bowl that is safe to microwave.

2. Add water and sprinkle with cinnamon.

3. Until tender, microwave on high for two to three minutes.

Total Time: 5 minutes; Cooking Time: 3 minutes;

Nutritional Value (per portion):

100 calories | Protein: nil | 26g of carbohydrates

Fat: 0 grams | 4g of fiber

7. Blueberry-Crunchy Soft-Cooked Oatmeal

Components:

- Half a cup of quick oats

- One cup of skim milk

- One-fourth cup blueberries

Guidelines:

1. Prepare the oats in milk as directed on the packet.

2. Add blueberries and toss to serve.

Total Time: 5 minutes Cooking Time: 5 minutes

Nutritional Value (per portion):

220 calories | 8g of protein | 35g of carbohydrates

4g of fat | 4g of fiber

8. Raisin-Rice Pudding

Components:

- One cup low-fat milk

- Two teaspoons of raisins

- Half a cup cooked white rice

- One spoonful of sugar

Guidelines:

1. Place rice and milk in a pot. Turn the heat to medium.

2. Add sugar and raisins and stir.

3. Simmer for ten minutes or until thickened. Serve hot or cold.

Cooking Time: 10 minutes

Nutritional Composition (per serving): 5 minutes

200 calories | 6g of protein | 35g of carbohydrates

4g of fat | 1g of fiber

9. Popsicles with Smoothies

Components:

- One cup of yogurt without fat

- 1/2 cup of mixed fruit, including berries and mango

- One tablespoon of honey

Guidelines:

1. Smoothly blend the fruit, yogurt, and honey.

2. Fill popsicle molds, then freeze for four hours or longer.

Cook Time: 4 hours of freezing Prep Time: 10 minutes

Nutritional Composition (per popsicle):

90 calories | 4g of protein | 15g of carbohydrates

Fat (2 grams) | 2g of fiber

10. Pureed Pumpkin, Softly Cooked

Components:

- One cup of pureed canned pumpkin and

- One tablespoon of honey

- Half a teaspoon of ground cinnamon

Guidelines:

1. Combine cinnamon, honey, and pumpkin puree.

2. You can serve it cold or heated.

Time to Prepare: 5 minutes; Time to Cook: 0 minutes

Nutritional Value (per portion):

150 calories | 1g of protein | 38g of carbohydrates

Fat: 0 grams | 4g of fiber

11. Ginger-Pear Compote Made with Soft Cooking

Components:

- 1/2 teaspoon ground ginger

- 1/4 cup water

- 2 ripe pears, peeled and chopped

Guidelines:

1. In a saucepan, mix the pears, water, and ginger.

2. Simmer for about ten minutes on low heat, or until pears are tender.

3. You can serve it cold or heated.

Cooking Time: 10 minutes

Nutritional Composition (per serving):

150 calories | Protein: nil | 38g of carbohydrates

Fat: 0 grams | 4g of fiber

12. Almonds and Honey with Vanilla Greek Yogurt

Components:

– 1/2 cup Greek yogurt with reduced fat

- One tablespoon of honey

- One tablespoon of almond slices

Guidelines:

1. Combine honey and Greek yogurt.

2. Add sliced almonds on top.

Time to Prepare: 5 minutes; Time to Cook: 0 minutes

Nutritional Value (per portion):

220 calories | 12g of protein | 30g of carbohydrates

8g of fat | 2g of fiber

13. Soft-Cooked Oat Cookies with Bananas

Components:

- Mashed one ripe banana

- Half a cup of quick oats

– 1/4 cup of raisins

Guidelines:

1. Set oven temperature to 175°C/350°F.

2. In a bowl, combine the banana, oats, and raisins.

3. Place heaping spoonfuls onto an oven tray.

4. Bake until firm, 10 to 12 minutes.

Time of Preparation: 10 minutes; Time of Cooking: 12 minutes; Nutritional Content (per cookie, single cookie): 80 calories | 2g of protein | 15g of carbohydrates Fat: 1 gram | 2g of fiber

14. Apple Cinnamon Muffins, Soft-Cooked

Components:

- 1/4 cup low-fat milk

- 1/2 cup applesauce

- 1 cup all-purpose flour

- One-fourth cup sugar

- One-half tsp baking powder

- Half a teaspoon of ground cinnamon

Guidelines:

1. Set oven temperature to 175°C/350°F.

2. In a bowl, combine flour, baking powder, and cinnamon.

3. Put the applesauce, milk, and sugar in another bowl.

4. Gently blend the wet and dry ingredients.

5. Fill muffin tins, bake for 15 to 20 minutes.

Time of Preparation: 10 minutes; Time of Cooking: 20 minutes; Nutritional makeup (per muffin):

150 calories | 3g of protein | 28g of carbohydrates

3g of fat | 1g of fiber

15. Strawberry Jelly Prepared Softly

Components:

- 1/4 cup water

- 1 cup pureed strawberries

- 2 tablespoons sugar

- 1 tablespoon gelatin powder

Guidelines:

1. In a saucepan, heat the water and sugar until they dissolve.

2. After adding the gelatin, turn off the heat.

3. Add pureed strawberries and stir.

4. Pour into molds and chill for approximately four hours, or until set.

Time of Preparation: 10 minutes; Time of Cooking: 5 minutes; Nutritional Make-Up (per Serving):
80 calories | 1g of protein | 20g of carbohydrates
Fat: 0 grams | 2g of fiber

These dishes offer a variety of satisfying snack and dessert options that are gentle on the stomach and appropriate for people who have gastroparesis. Depending on your tolerance and tastes, change the components and quantity sizes.

CONCLUSION

Now that we've completed our adventure through the "Gastroparesis Cookbook for Beginners," it's important to take stock of the insightful knowledge and useful tips we've gained. Because gastroparesis presents certain difficulties, meal preparation and planning must be done with caution. With the help of this cookbook, we hope to give you a solid foundation of recipes that satisfy your cravings for comfort, variety, and satisfaction while also meeting the nutritional requirements of those who have gastroparesis.

With its delayed stomach emptying, gastroparesis can have a significant influence on day-to-day living. Abdominal pain, bloating, nausea, and vomiting are some of the symptoms that the illness may produce. Gout management necessitates more than just modifying meal portions; it frequently entails substantial alterations to the kinds of foods eaten, how they are prepared, and how they are consumed. Reducing symptoms and meeting nutritional needs are the main objectives.

It is important to comprehend these dietary requirements. Generally speaking, foods that are readily digested, low in fat, and moderately high in fiber are advised. Foods with smooth textures, low fat content, and low fiber content facilitate digestion and lessen the strain on the stomach. With a variety of recipes tailored to these requirements, this cookbook makes navigating gastroparesis both much tastier and somewhat more doable.

The Significance of a Balanced Diet

Making sure your diet is balanced is one of the most important parts of managing gastroparesis. Eating habits are equally as important as the food you consume. Every cuisine in this book is designed to be easy on the stomach and yet deliver vital nutrients. These meals are designed to keep you full and nourished, from energizing breakfast choices to hearty dinners and filling snacks.

A thoughtful selection of nutrient-dense and easily digestible ingredients is how balance is created. This cookbook includes mainstays like boiled veggies, low-fat dairy products, and lean proteins like chicken and fish. These nutrients support the body's need for vitamins and minerals without overburdening the digestive tract.

Accepting Diverseness and Originality

Flavor and diversity are not sacrificed in the name of managing gastroparesis. This cookbook proves that having dietary limitations doesn't have to prevent you from enjoying a wide variety of dishes. These recipes are meant to be flexible and adaptive. Everything from refreshing smoothies to hearty bowls of soft-cooked oats can be found here to suit every taste and preference.

You can give your dishes a new twist without bothering your stomach by experimenting with milder herbs and spices. The progressive introduction of new flavors and textures might help the dietary shift go more smoothly and enjoyably for people who are apprehensive about trying new ingredients.

Useful Advice for Efficient Meal Planning

A key component of controlling gastroparesis is efficient meal preparation. The following useful advice will assist you in navigating your food journey:

1. Make a plan ahead: Making meals ahead of time can guarantee that you always have gastroparesis-friendly options available and will also help to reduce the stress associated with preparing at the last minute.

2. Small, Frequent Meals: Throughout the day, eating more often and in smaller portions will help control symptoms and enhance digestion.

3. Maintain Hydration: It can be beneficial to drink fluids in between meals as opposed to with them to avoid feeling full and bloated.

4. Monitor Tolerance: Track the effects of various foods on your symptoms. Since everyone has a different tolerance, it's critical to customize your diet to suit your needs.

5. Speak with Experts: Consulting with a dietician or other healthcare professional can assist address unique nutritional needs and offer individualized guidance.

The Strength of Support and Community

Although having gastroparesis can occasionally make you feel alone, you are not. Participating in support groups, whether they be online or in person, can offer shared experiences, practical guidance, and emotional support. These groups can provide support, recipe exchanges, and coping mechanisms that can greatly improve your condition management.

It can be really fulfilling to share recipes and your personal experiences with others. You can assist others in navigating their dietary issues and finding solace in the knowledge that they are part of a supportive network by adding to the larger dialogue on gastroparesis.

It is important to keep in mind that managing gastroparesis is a continuous process as you experiment and modify the recipes within this cookbook. It entails ongoing education, flexibility, and self-care. These recipes are meant to serve as a starting point; they offer a range of possibilities that may be adjusted to meet your dietary requirements and personal tastes.

You can manage gastroparesis more easily and enjoyably by including these recipes into your regular routine. Accept the process, pay attention to your body, and modify as necessary. Finding the diet that works best for you will improve your health and enable you to live a more comfortable lifestyle. Your dietary journey is unique.

The "Gastroparesis Cookbook for Beginners" is a resource that aims to provide you with the knowledge and useful tools you need to effectively manage your illness; it's not just a cookbook. This cookbook attempts to assist you in your pursuit of a well-balanced and pleasurable diet by offering mild, nourishing, and tasty meal options.

Remember that each meal is an opportunity to fuel yourself and adopt a healthier, more manageable lifestyle when you put this book down and begin your culinary adventure. I hope this cookbook is a useful resource, an inspiration, and proof that you can still have tasty, fulfilling meals even when you have dietary limitations.